Training Your Body For Life

A Simple Guide For Muscle and Health

by Michael LaPlante

© Author 2019

Edition 1

Table of Contents

Who Should Read This Guide?

I wrote this for the man or woman who may have spent time in the gym, or track, or ball field while in their teens and twenties, but who has settled for the idea that maturing and growing into middle age, say thirty five or forty and beyond, means that an increase in body weight, decrease in flexibility, aches and pains and a general loss of physical function are normal and to be expected. They are not, and I want to implore and encourage you to begin to think in terms of functional strength and flexibility as goals which are relatively easy to accomplish, as long as you start slow and keep things ridiculously simple.

You can do this! Even if you have physical limitations, a previous injury that never quite healed, you work crazy hours and have too many demands on your time, you will benefit from the advice in this book. Hell, the crazier and busier your life is, the more this book will help you on your journey. I have been there, I have fought the demons and I know what works and doesn't for me, and I want you to benefit from my experiences with fitness and health so you can live your life free from chronic pain, illness, medications and all the suffering that goes along with that.

Investing a small amount of time and thought on your number one asset, your health, will pay you back a thousand-fold. You must not give in to conventional wisdom which is both untrue and unwise. You can have a better functioning body at any age. You can feel and perform better and with less pain!

There was a time when I wouldn't be caught dead training with anything other than free weights. Sure, I had used various resistance machines and at one point even owned a heavy weight stack machine, a Soloflex resistance band machine, and other devices such as incline rower, flex bands, treadmill and such. But free weights were, for a young man of 20 or so, the ultimate challenge. I found that once I progressed to a moderately conditioned state, which meant that the weight I was using increased, it was plain for all to see who was the real hoss in the room. I had good natural functional strength and loved things like rope climbing, which I could accomplish easily, even without the help of my legs and feet gripping the rope.

But my goal back then was not functional strength at all, it was all about being attractive to women. Yes, working out for reasons of vanity is, as most eventually learn, silly and even dangerous. Taken to the extreme, with steroids and insane dietary routines, barbell training and the whole body building genre are traps many young people, mostly men, fall into and then struggle mightily to escape.

I am lucky, while I pushed myself with weight training, and I over-trained often to the point of soreness and even light muscle tearing and straining, that I avoided long term problems that are common to the sport. By problems I mean pain. Pain is, I have learned, something you build up and collect over time, like a savings account with a horrible interest rate. It has taken me the better part of 60 years, but I now have pain that visits on a daily basis, usually for brief periods, in my Achilles tendons, a very old muscle tear in my back, two fingers I jammed repeatedly and so forth.

Earlier this year, out of nowhere, I began to feel neuropathy in my lower right leg, likely from something called mast cell activation. What a hoot that is! It is an intense burning deep inside the limb, and the cool part is, when you reflexively rub or massage the area, it gets much, much worse. Then suddenly, usually after 10 or 15 minutes, poof – gone. I entered Army boot camp as a young man sporting two sprained ankles I got while training, ironically, to prepare for boot camp. I ran daily in heavy gear despite the pain and swelling and somehow made it through an extended 6 month training regimen in that condition. Is this finally coming back to haunt some thirty five years later?

Point is, we appear to heal from our injuries, but, surprise! Somehow even long forgotten traumas will re-emerge as we grow older. I have no clue why this is. I suppose things like entropy, hormone levels, weakening immune system, genetics, possibly ex-spouses and who knows what else are factors here. I do know that a portion of the pain I carry daily is directly due to abusing myself in the gym thirty or so years ago. The body never forgets.

If you find anything at all in this guide that helps you, please know that your comment on Amazon will go a long way to help spread the word. It is said a lot and lacks apparent sincerely, but I am truly grateful for your time. ***Thank you.***

Forty is the old age of youth; fifty the youth of old age. - Victor Hugo

Body weight Resistance Training Exercises

Contrary to popular belief, lifting heavy weights repeatedly to stimulate muscle hypertrophy is completely pointless unless your goal is to be the next Mister or Miss Universe. In that case by all means, go for it. Know that the elite body-builders are often among the most doped-up and unhealthy people on the planet. Many die young from this insane beauty contest sometimes referred to as a sport. You want to be buff to be attractive to the opposite sex? Sure, I get that. But this may also be misguided when you look at the top traits your future partner finds most appealing.

According to Askmen.com, having bulging muscles or looking like a gym-stud doesn't even make the top ten list of qualities women look for in a man. In fact, everything women mention as being attractive have to do with personality, with humor as the number one most important quality. Sure, there are some women who get turned on by the body-builder physic, but I would bet that even the members of that group value personality and humor as important or critical to any future relationship with you.

For their part, men rank bodily attractiveness of women as number six in their top ten most important list. Things like empathy, ability to listen and being self-sacrificing all rated higher than her pure physical characteristics. Granted, three of the top ten were physical traits; facial appearance, waist to hip ratio, and body attractiveness, but being buff or ripped are nowhere to be found whereas having an attractive face, eyes and mouth are high on the list for men.

It should be obvious that the time spent grinding out double split sets and two per day gym visits, lat and calf day and all the other gravity fighting stuff you may have been doing, amounts to basically hard, manual labor with very little payoff in terms of attracting the opposite sex, health, or personal development and so forth. Understand that your physical appearance and health are critical. Like so many other things I talk about, the trick is balance and overall benefit, not just biceps measurements.

What you really need is functional conditioning and flexibility, and body-weight resistance training is how you achieve and maintain it, throughout your life.

When you use your own body and gravity instead of iron plates or machines, you exercise in a recoverable way and over time, build up your entire system. You also avoid working on a specific muscle or limited muscle group, which is likely with barbells and machines. Isolation exercises are a wasteful tax on your energy and recovery and we have no time for this!

We move muscle systems when working and playing, not isolated muscle. Causing hypertrophy or growth by basically damaging one muscle at a time and then waiting for the body to repair it is potentially harmful. It also makes you a slave to the process, which is fine if you have the time and are realizing a personal passion through body-building. Otherwise, it is a misguided approach to exercise, and I would beg you to approach your gym or workout from another direction entirely.

The best part of body weight resistance training is how good it makes you feel. You are, by design, working your body as a single unit. Muscle soreness and over training are mostly eliminated by the fact that it is so much more difficult to over train your body when your exercise involves multiple muscle groups than when isolating, (and abusing), an individual muscle.

I remember reading the muscle magazines in the 1980's and kept bumping into concepts such as this: If you want bigger arms, train your legs. Looking for more defined abdominals, do more squats and so forth. It was out of the box thinking at the time, but it points to the heart of the matter which is that the biggest benefit we can derive from resistance training is by using the biggest and most muscle possible at any one time. This is timeless advice, now all we need is a healthy replacement for iron bars and weight stacks that tear muscle and break down our bodies.

The following three exercises are best when they form the core of your workout routine. They are easy to begin with and learn but are extremely difficult to master. They will work all your muscles intensely, and should be done in order. You want to be slow and brief with these in the beginning and let your system get used to this new assault. The point is to allow your body to adapt over time. You will know when the time has come to increase the reps, decrease the interval between exercises and otherwise up the intensity. Within a couple months, depending on how you feel, you should build up to three brief sessions per week. Monday, Wednesday, Friday is ideal. I always feel more energetic when well rested between workouts, and brief but vigorous sessions are vastly superior to grinding out set after set, like hard labor that tears you down and eventually destroys your motivation.

Remember, exercise is a privilege in which many people cannot participate. The goal should always be to enjoy the benefits provided by exercise: flexibility, energy, vitality etc, rather than exercise for its own sake, or vanity, ego and the like. You want the briefest workout possible that provides beneficial stress on your body. Your gains in physical and mental abilities occur during the rest periods when you are recovering. There will be days when you are sore or tired or lack sleep for whatever reason. Skip your workout and rest! Live to fight another day as it were. We seek gradual, sustainable improvement over a lifetime, not 'big guns in 6 weeks', or whatever B.S. is being sold this month. Here is the core workout:

The Body weight Squat

This is basically a standing squat done with strict form and it works your entire system including your lung power. It looks easy, and knocking out five or ten is no huge deal. Fifty in a row will feel like you sprinted a 10K, and you will want to build up slowly to that number. Ultimately, you will condition yourself to perform 100 - 150 without stopping. At that level, you are truly in good functional condition and will enjoy the challenge. Your breathing during this is the most important aspect of the exercise.

- Stand with feet slightly apart with arms extended straight out in front

- Pull your arms in a strong rowing motion inward as you fully inhale

- Slowly lower yourself toward the floor, going as low as comfortably possible, as you exhale

- As you move down, your arms are also moving down and behind your body.

- Without stopping at the bottom, swing your arms upward and back out as you rise up and inhale

- Back to standing position, your arms are again extended and you flow right into the next rowing motion

- Vary the movement by keeping the heels on the floor or let them rise up as you move up and down.

- Remember to fully exhale while moving downward and inhale while rising up. This seems backwards at first. Done properly, this requires a full, controlled inhale and exhale that you will learn to coordinate with your up and down motion

Once you get the hang of this exercise if will become very fluid and you can concentrate on a continuous motion and your breathing. You don't want to be stopping and 'gathering yourself' during this exercise. Keep your muscles under tension and focus on being smooth and balanced. Start with five or less if you have to. Let your body decide when to progress. The point is to start and this is a wonderful place to begin.

The Mountain Push-up

After a brief rest and partial recovery from the squats, no more than 5 minutes, but perhaps more in the beginning, you want to launch into the Mountain Push-up. This is another total body exercise, and form and breathing are critical. This movement builds serious upper body strength in the chest and shoulders, and also targets spine and hip flexibility. Done correctly it is also a beast. Shoot for 1 to 5 controlled, full reps in the beginning. When you are able to execute 20 to 25, you are quite the bad ass!

- Assume push-up position, however your hips are raised and back is straight, like an inverted 'V' or mountain. Feet are wider than shoulders, head is down.

- Simultaneously move hips down and forward as you move elbows out, keep driving forward and as you draw elbows back in. You are moving in a big serpentine arc with your body, ending with hips down, head and shoulders raised up. Feet still apart. I like to focus on the path my head is taking and my body follows like a big snake. Practice fluid, smooth, controlled movement. Big inhale while still looking up.

- Reverse the movement, pressing backward while raising your hips and stretching your legs, ending again in the inverted 'V' with head down. You will feel the intensity in your upper body. Exhale. (I usually begin the next rep sometime during the exhale).

- Knock out as many as you can comfortably. Be especially careful in the beginning and let your shoulders get used to this.

The Mountain Climber

Another brief rest and then one final assault on the entire body and breathing. Starting position is similar to Mountain Push-up, but as you begin, you hips and back will be more or less level with the floor while you execute a running movement by alternately bringing left and right feet and legs forward towards each elbow. No stopping allowed, just basically running while your hands remain in a wide, push-up position contact with the floor. Breathe deeply throughout the exercise and build up over time with a target of 120 and above repetitions.

- Push-up position, hips slightly elevated. Feet wide but balanced so you can start to 'run'

- Alternate bringing one foot forward as far as possible, then while moving it back to start position, the other leg is simultaneously moving forward. Other words, legs are both in constant motion throughout.

- I like to focus on pointing my knees forward and back in a fluid motion.

- Don't forget to breathe deeply throughout.

This is a great finishing exercise and you will feel fairly wiped out in the beginning. With time, after a brief rest you will feel exhilarated and ready to take on the planet, which is the idea!

What About the Warm-up?

This might sound strange to you, but except for brief, light stretching, usually just a couple of careful neck stretches and maybe a torso and hamstring stretch, mostly to get my head in the game, the exercises themselves are the best warm-up that could possibly exist. This is another distinct advantage of body weight resistance training - the time commitment is significantly reduced.

It makes sense if you think about it. How do you best warm up for body weight squats or mountain push-ups? By doing them! Here is the thing to focus on: you are performing a single, maxed out set of each exercise, 3 days per week. None of the movements, performed with strict form, are destructive to the body, and the threat of over training is zero. Time spent warming up becomes largely unproductive and wasteful. Besides, if you find yourself warming up a muscle group to overcome soreness, perhaps you should be resting anyway, and not exercising?

You might want to get your heart rate and breathing up a bit before diving into these, if that helps you mentally get going. But remember, as you perform the movements you are taking full breaths and moving in a controlled, slow, manor. Your body will quickly warm up, trust me on this.

The final analysis here is that I have never injured myself doing body weight movements, while I have injured myself with weights, despite protracted warming up. The choice, and results, are yours. Do what feels best to you.

My 3 Alternate Exercises

The three exercises above are really all you ever need to maintain and improve your strength and flexibility throughout your life. I will admit, however, that there are times when the need for variety strikes and I find myself looking forward to alternate exercises to keep things interesting, and myself motivated. A few years ago I found a body weight gym on Craigslist and set it up in my shop. It quickly became indispensable and is one of only three pieces of equipment I believe everyone should own. The others will be discussed in later chapters. **Note: the body weight gym is not required for the alternate exercises**, but is a nice-to-have item for the long haul.

The one pictured below is nearly identical to mine and was for sale on Ebay for less than $200 at the time I was writing this book. It features stations for: the pullup, pushup, dips, and abdominals. It does not address the leg muscles, however, the body weight squat is a superb way to warm up and prime your system for the exercises performed on this gym.

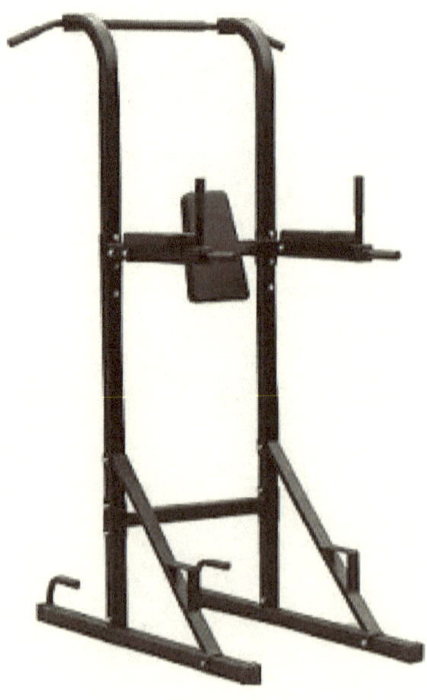

Alternate Exercise One - The Push-up

The humble push-up, done correctly is a great upper body workout because of all the muscles groups it involves. Correct form with these, and really every exercise, involves constant tension with absolutely no stopping or 'locking out' at either the top or bottom of the movement. You want to think about a single, 60 or 90 second repetition, which involves 10 or 20 or whatever you can perform, up and down components, rather than individual reps that you count out with pauses in between. Actually, the slower you go, and thus the fewer reps you do, the better! Think about it, imagine a single rep that takes 5 minutes from start to finish. The strongest and fittest person on Earth would likely have great difficulty performing one.

The point is, it matters little how many you do, it's the intensity you apply to doing them that matters. Go very slow, don't stop or lock out, and give it your all until failure and move on until next time. Do the pushup on the body weight gym for a bit more extension at the bottom and benefit from even more intensity.

Push-up Variation #1 - The Plank

Sometimes I will perform a few slow pushups and actually stop at the top of the movement and hold that position until failure. This is normally referred to as the Plank. The Plank works surprisingly well as a full body exercise, and you really feel it in your core. Remember to never lock your elbows, so your weight stays on the muscles rather than the joints. As you approach failure, you may lock elbows to cheat out some additional time in position. Done right, you will appreciate this sneaky-tough exercise.

Push-up Variation #2 - The Dip

The Dip requires the body weight gym or some other parallel bar type construct you put together in your garage or property. I have read about Dip-devotees who do nothing else besides Dips and Squats and they sport enviable physiques. There was a time when I could pound out 3 sets of 25 or more, with good form. These days, I Dip for variety and I notice that they isolate the shoulder a little too much for my tastes, so caution is advised. The beauty of the Dip is that by holding your legs either forward or behind your torso you significantly change the exercise and its degree of difficulty. Try to vary your position slowly during the set. Start with knees pulled up, which is really tough, and as you slowly move up and down - no locking out - bring your legs down and then pull your feet up behind your body. This moves your weight and angle of attack from front to back and demolishes your shoulder/chest/upper back muscles. Failure comes quickly when done right.

I like to start in the up or arms-extended position, then I draw may knees up and forward, making a sort of 'J' shape with my body, then slowly and smoothly lower myself until I feel a good stretch across my chest and shoulders, and without stopping at the bottom begin to press back up. Without locking out at the top I begin the downward motion for a second time etc. Remember, as you get used to this exercise, try holding your feet up behind you and carefully experiment with the 'J' shape to change the angle of your dips. Avoid leaning too far forward and isolating the pectoral muscles. Keep your chin tucked into your chest. Good luck.

Alternate Exercise Two - The Pull-up

Another superb total body exercise, the pull-up, is also commonly attempted with poor form and thus turned into somewhat of an isolation exercise, which is unfortunate. The reason this happens is that a single rep is quite difficult or even impossible for most people so in exchange for a repetition correct form is assassinated. This is understandable because, after all, we humans have engineered our surroundings in such a way that the need for pulling, gripping and swinging are in low demand, and our aptitude in these areas is low.

Practice the Pull-up by using a stool or other platform so that you can keep your back straight and head down, and pull with your upper body as you assist with your legs. Try to hold at the top with the bar touching the back of your neck, then lift your legs and just hold the position as long as possible, even as you begin to fail and slowly, but in a controlled way, fall into the arms extended position. You can even start at the top of the movement and execute a **Reverse Pull-up**, which is especially helpful in the beginning.

Focus your mind on your back rather than your arms and you will gain significant strength over time by doing these with a chair or stool-assist. Picture your shoulder blades moving towards the center of your back as you pull. As always, form and intensity provide the value here, not the number of reps.

Alternate Exercise Three - The Belly Burner

Dumb name I will admit, but a great mid-section workout. I remember reading about it thirty years ago, tried it, and couldn't believe how crazy well it worked my abdominals and back, the muscle groups that are so important for posture and core strength. Most exercises that target them are a literal waste of time and energy and, like the situp, are potentially harmful to your hard tissue. If you want six-pack abs, do more squats and cardio and eat fewer calories, period. For conditioning and core strength, and overall toning, we have the Belly Burner!

Begin in a standing position with your feet shoulder width apart, hands on hips. Now, as you begin to exhale, bend forward at the waist as far as possible while maintaining good balance. Your goal is to completely force the air from your lungs, and your bending and diaphragm squeezing is helping you do this.

Great, so now you are fully bent over forward and have forced every ounce of air from your lungs, you are holding a big squeeze with your abdominals. Now begin to raise your torso back to vertical, but without breathing in! As you straighten back up, you also maintain your ab-squeeze, and concentrate on lifting your chest, as hard as you can, toward the ceiling. Done correctly, you will feel a very intense muscle tension throughout your abdomen and all the way around your lower and even mid-back. Hold the upper position with chest high for as long as you can, then rest. Repeat this after a brief rest, perhaps once or twice, but be careful in the beginning as you are working muscles and groups that likely have not been worked in quite awhile. This one is special, as you will discover. Enjoy!

Abdominal Variation - Body weight Gym Ab-Station

One of the nice features of the gym is its ab-station, and the way it stabilizes the torso while you basically do leg-lifts with squeezing of the abdominals. Since this movement involves the arms and shoulders for stabilization, plus core and hip muscles, it really is a great total body exercise.

Start with your elbows on the horizontal pads, hands gripping the handle-bars and your back up against the long, vertical pad. Your feet are dangling in the air because your weight is being supported by your hands, forearms and elbows. Now, bring knees up as high as you can while squeezing your abdominals, hold briefly at the top and then slowly lower knees back to near starting position. Do not relax at the bottom; you want to keep the abdominals under tension throughout the exercise. Do as many slow repetitions as you can, one set, then move on.

The gym pad forces you to use good form which makes this exercise more difficult than it appears. You are also prevented from arching your back while lifting your knees, and as with all exercise, going slow provides the true win-win of being both safer and more intense at the same time.

As you improve on the ab-station, try bringing up your knees slightly to the left of center, then center, then right of center as you execute your controlled repetitions.

The goal here is to work the entire mid-section, so concentrate on flexing your working muscles, from front to back as you perform this.

Honorable Mention - The Easy Bridge

This exercise deserves to be on your short list for several reasons. The Easy Bridge can be performed in place of the Mountain Pushup, especially in the beginning when you are more likely to experience a little soreness from the previous session. It also contracts and or stretches all the major muscle groups simultaneously, and, like the plank is a great finishing exercise.

Despite the name, this is anything but easy and you want to be careful because of the uniqueness of the demands this places on your muscles and connective tissue.

- Start in a crouched position and lean back on both hands to stabilize your body.

- Now lift up your hips as you adjust both feet and hands to form a table with your body. Face points up toward the ceiling.

- Focus on body position, arms are straight with elbows locked, legs bent at the knee, body is held as level as possible. You are a human coffee table at this point.

- Feel your back, glutes and hamstrings contracting to support this position, while chest, shoulders and arms stretch.

- Hold as long as you can, then slowly sit down on the floor and rest.

Think of everyone you will run into today and how few of them would be able to pull off the Easy Bridge. We never want to be in that group!

Conclusion

These resistance exercises are all you need for life to improve and maintain whatever level of conditioning you desire. Every large muscle group is addressed, and most work on multiple groups simultaneously. Remember to focus on brief, intense workouts that allow your body time to rest and recover. There is enough variation here to keep you challenged and interested while your system improves and adapts to the new physical demands you are placing on it.

Often, life will get in the way and prevent you from exercising on a day you had planned to do so. So what! Let your system benefit from a longer rest and you will approach the next workout with even more enthusiasm.

One huge benefit of body weight resistance training is the ability to workout wherever you happen to be; hotel room, office, guest room at your in-laws, etc. By removing the usual obstacles to exercising such as traveling to a gym, workout clothes and supplies, membership fees, time, and so forth, you begin to realize how easy it is to fit a workout in to your weekly routine. There is literally nothing stopping you!

How To Revive a Fish aka Heart Health

One of the most interesting medical doctors I ever met was Dr. Kim, a South Korean and graduate of the Tokyo School of Medicine. A quick story to give you an idea why; during an early, general discussion about the field of medicine, Dr Kim asked me what I thought was the most important drug ever created. "Penicillin" was my quick answer. "Milk of Magnesia", he said with a smile. He was quite serious too. He advised all his patients to take a spoonful in a glass of water every morning, and again a half hour before dinner. He believed that keeping the Gastrointestinal tract healthy was the key to good health, and this was how you went about it. Funny how that information stuck with me after probably twenty years. No, I don't follow that advice although I would bet Dr. Kim still does and would also not be surprised if he was still a top athlete and martial artist.

Another occasion Dr Kim was talking about heart health and how it relates to leg and lung power. His point was that the legs are a vital part of our circulatory system design and without them, our heart muscle would have to be much larger to move all the blood our bodies require for optimum health. He taught that by conditioning the legs, pressure or stress is taken off the heart and we are healthier overall.

"How do you revive a nearly dead fish?", he was ask. "By holding it in the water and gently moving its tail back and forth". His point was that the back and forth movement of the tail was a life-giving motion because it helped its heart and lungs pump oxygen throughout its body and brain. Our legs provide the same benefit to us, he would say. It certainly sounds plausible to me. Where am I going with this? Glad you asked, read on.

Aerobic Training

There are times when I just don't feel like resistance training, for no good reason other than boredom or laziness. Aerobic training is difficult for me because I find walking as an exercise incredibly boring, and running even worse; boring yet destructive to the joints, (Please, no hate mail). Besides, with few exceptions, when have you looked at a long distance runner's body and thought, "Boy, that's the physique I'm looking for!" I never have. Runners just look emaciated and worn, despite their incredible abilities. I will admit I could be dead wrong about distance running for conditioning. It may be the best single thing for the body for all I know. I do believe that sprinting in intervals, that is to say, brief but hard running, resting, then hard running again, resting, etc, is fantastic exercise. Sprinters appear to have impressive and muscular physiques. Personally, it just isn't for me.

Bicycling - Because Hello, The Wheel Was Invented!

So, as I was saying, on those days where I just don't feel like resistance training, which, when done properly, provides incredible aerobic training in its own right, I will instead turn to my bicycle. I strongly recommend that you get a bike if you can and it is the second of the three supplemental pieces of fitness equipment I own and think you should too.

The problem a lot of people have with bicycling, especially those suffering from any kind of arm or shoulder pain, arthritis and really any upper body issue, is the riding position required by bicycles. This is because most bikes position the rider over the handlebars with weight somewhat forward, and this places a good deal of stress on the arms, hands and wrists. This causes soreness and becomes the main limiting factor to the length and benefit of the ride.

Introducing the modified recumbent bicycle.

A few years ago I stumbled upon a bike made by a company called Day 6, that addresses the weight-forward problems associated with most bicycles, and I instantly had to have one. This one is almost identical to mine and I found it on Craigslist for $450, which is a good average used price for these.

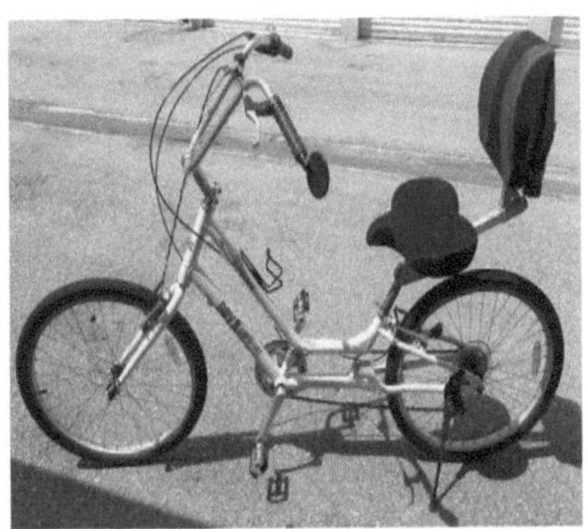

The Day 6 design moves the rider's weight back behind the pedals and against its over-sized seat and back rest. The handle bars reach back to the rider, rather than forcing the rider to reach forward for the bars. This eliminates the pressure on the hands, wrists and arms and also affords maximum torque to be applied to the pedals. One of the very first rides I took on mine was when I loaded it in the car and drove to the bike trail and, with no practice or build-up rode for just under 40 miles, with a brief 5 minute rest at the turn-around for a bathroom and water break. This was during summer in Florida and I recovered quickly and was not sore the next day. My legs felt slightly rubbery because of the extra workout, but it was a good kind of non-destructive post workout sensation.

Previously, I owned a more typical Canondale bike and I would start to fatigue across my neck and shoulders after about 12 - 13 miles and call it a workout. I had no idea at the time how important riding position is to performance. The light bulb came on, so to speak, when the Day 6 showed me that wrist and shoulder fatigue are unnecessary and avoidable on a bicycle. The aerobic potential in a properly designed bike is phenomenal. Since I'm not racing, I don't need aerodynamics. I ride for conditioning and this is, for me, the perfect aerobic exercise, bar none.

There are other modified as well as full recumbent bicycles out there. Craigslist and Ebay frequently carry them. Even if you have a traditional bike and are comfortable on it, that's great! Get your legs moving, lungs working and heartbeat elevated for 30 minutes or so on the days when you are taking a break from the other stuff. Think of reviving that fish and keep your legs moving soldier!

Smokers are People Too

I sympathize with smokers and the crap they endure for it. Possibly because I have been there. I believe that most things in moderation are fine, including smoking. I also believe that switching to cigar or pipe smoking is beneficial because of the problems associated with inhaling the combustibles from the paper used to wrap cigarettes. That said, smokers may benefit from increased aerobic training, such as bicycling or walking, and may even find that those exercises lengthen the time interval between their desire to light up the next cigarette. Assuming the evidence is correct, that smoking adds to arterial plaque, reduces oxygenation - including to the brain, and also dries out your system, this suggests to me that a healthy diet and aerobic exercise along with extra water intake are potentially offsetting activities and distinctly benefit those who wish to smoke.

Smoking is obviously a personal choice. If you do smoke, enjoy it but limit it. If you love French fries, same exact thing applies. In either case, focus on aerobic activity and maximize your lung power training with the squat and bicycle or walking.

If you want to quit but still smoke, then you don't want to quit. Perhaps you should just limit your consumption to a certain quantity per day and work with that. Some believe it is the tobacco companies who espouse the idea that nicotine is more addictive than heroin. Their contention is that it is actually easy to quit, we've just been manipulated to think otherwise. Hey, sugar is addictive too and yet there are no doubt excessive sugar-eaters out there who also denigrate smokers. The point is, I have found that anything in moderation, exercise included, that does not hurt someone else, is fine if you enjoy it. Otherwise, worrying about it is pointless.

When you're really ready to quit, you will, and you will feel crappy for awhile but then better after that. Exercising is a great way to overcome the after-affects of quitting, as well as the affects of smoking. Your choice either way. Embrace it and move on.

Exercises For Better Vision - Are Glasses Optional?

I had perfect eyesight until I reached my early forties, then suddenly one day, I remember being in some big store, likely a grocery store, and I had difficulty reading the small print on the labels. That was a bummer because it was for me a sort of aging wake-up call, as if I needed another one besides the reflection in my mirror!

Most, if not all training books out there completely overlook this most important sensory organ which is unfortunate. Basically speaking, our eyes are amazing visible light focus machines. As we age, our natural ability to place the image of the object we are looking at onto a specific piece of real estate at the back of the eyeball diminishes. Sadly, the first thing we do is run to the store to purchase reading glasses to compensate for this. From then on it becomes a game of coping with and adjusting to an ever changing field of vision and the corrective lenses that serve to delay the inevitable. I stubbornly refuse to get contact lenses, and until our medical establishment progresses beyond the pre-modern era in which it is mired, nobody is pointing a laser at my eyes. There must be something else we can do to limit or even correct our vision problems!

Some of you may already be familiar with Dr. William Bates 1860 - 1931, who was an American ophthalmologist and developer of the **Bates Method** and author of the 1920 book, ***Perfect Sight Without Glasses***. Dr. Bate's methodology was, and is controversial, as are most iconoclasts and mavericks. Dr. Bates believed that glasses are actually damaging to the eyes and he developed a series of exercises, stretches and relaxation techniques to train the eyes and restore their ability to focus.

The point is, there exist long held points of view that are different than the established routine of heading to Lenscrafters as soon as our vision goes south. It behooves us all to learn about the choices and alternatives available, and thus make better decisions. It is important to know that it is possible to exercise the muscles surrounding the eyeball, and thus manipulate its shape which basically repositions the area at the back of the eye relative to the focal point of the image being placed there, thereby bringing it into focus. We see with our brains, not our eyes. The object or landscape we are staring at is right there (although upside down) inside our eyeball, nice and clear. We just need to strengthen the muscles that allow us to change the shape of our eyeball so that the image lands right on the patch in the back. Simple, right?

Exercises that have helped me have names such as sunning, palming, swaying etc. And Bates used a lot of visualization and relaxation techniques to train the eyes, connect the two brain hemispheres and so forth.

One interesting exercise covered in the video link below entails placing hands over the eyes to block light otherwise coming through the eyelids, and concentrating on seeing pure, pitch black. The example given is to think about a black piano, and that helps, also my phone is shiny black etc. It is more difficult than it sounds, especially when I do that right after the Sunning exercise. Trying to hold the image of jet-black for more than a couple seconds is surprisingly difficult. It made me realize that seeing certain things is more of a mental construct that can actually be practiced and improved upon. There are several others, but the point is, I notice improvement when I do these and I want you to check out the links below, as well as others you find, (I have zero affiliation with them), and take from it what works for you.

A most excellent website I found that is based on the teaching of Dr. Bates is here: http://www.seeing.org/techniques/ and I urge you to spend some time checking it out, even if you are a natural skeptic. There are actually many websites and YouTube videos that discuss and demonstrate his methods. Here is an example of a YouTube lecture about it: https://www.youtube.com/watch?v=TbMze4Ok6Ns

If the link changes or otherwise becomes unavailable, just search YouTube and/or Wikipedia for Dr. William H. Bates, which currently is right here: https://en.wikipedia.org/wiki/William_Bates_(physician) ...you will no doubt find his information.

What if Dr. Bates is correct and worsening eyesight does not have to be an accepted fact of aging? I think it's worth looking into.

Eating Right is a P.I.T.A.

Diet is one of those things that is so personal and complicated that we all fall into patterns of unhealthy eating for convenience and out of habit which, over time, cause lots of unintended consequences. I am as guilty of this as the next poor soul.

I have conditioned myself to make food and meal choices in terms of, 'What would my grandparents do?" Strange, yes, but it provides me an easy gauge to apply to this area. My grandparents, whom I miss dearly, were born in the early 1900's and thus were just about my current age before fast food and highly processed and preserved food were invented. They spent more time and effort acquiring and preparing food, but it was less adulterated with chemicals and hormones, had a much shorter shelf-life, and was healthier overall.

They ate the food that our illustrious medical establishment would later warn us not to eat: eggs, coffee, butter, red meat, etc. and instead we were told that man-made, low fat, artificially sweetened, processed food was better for us. So we listened and so began the national obesity epidemic that rages to this day.

What works for me and my metabolism may be disastrous for you. However, I believe that we should all keep a few things in mind when it comes to eating, and use my grandparents to guide us. I have been eating the way I do for so long that I am rarely even tempted by the bad stuff, except that I do have a weakness for salty snacks, especially when driving, (my wife says I should keep a salt lick in my car). Here are the guidelines I follow. I rarely get sick and even when I do, I have not missed a day of work in 30 years, so it is safe to say at the very least, my diet is likely not holding me back.

Here are the foods that are important to my diet:

- I try to consume 2 or 3 eggs each and every day - I consider these my multi-vitamin, multi-mineral supplement. Organic, free range eggs are relatively inexpensive these days. Learn to love eggs. Lightly scrambled or soft-boiled eggs take just a few minutes to prepare.

- Black coffee, a single, very strong cup in the morning. No sugar, sometimes I add butter for flavor

- Fruit - I especially like apples, and bananas, but only in the morning

- Salad - with dinner, various ingredients including mushrooms, natural olives, and with olive oil and apple cider vinegar dressing or healthy alternatives

- Protein - wild caught fish whenever possible, grass fed beef, chicken. I try to limit meat consumption because too much is a workout for the kidneys. I find that I don't need as much as I did twenty plus years ago anyway

- Peanuts and peanut butter is good food, look for natural, additive free PB.

- Nuts – definitely but in moderation. Almonds are great but can cause me G.I. trouble.

- Drink - I normally have spring water with me, I like carbonated water too. I tend to put some kind of electrolyte in it for flavor and health reasons. Florida's heat & humidity will wear you right out if you work outside and neglect fluids. Also, I avoid flooding my system with water when eating to allow my stomach acid to better break down my food.

- I try to wait until noon to eat anything except fruit, and I rarely eat anything at all after 8pm. The body needs rest!

- Beer, wine, spirits - everything in moderation. I usually wait for the weekend and enjoy a couple drinks with zero guilt. If I am with friends and playing guitar, I drink more beer. It's liquid bread so shoot me.

Things on my prohibited list - these are things that I cut out of my diet years ago, and the weird part I found is that I never crave any of it. Take sugar as an example. Highly refined sugar is in everything and it is unhealthy, leeches vitamins and minerals from you body, rots teeth, feeds bad bacteria, yadda, yadda. Small doses I'm sure are fine, but people crave sugar for whatever reason and that fact alone makes me wary and careful with it.

A few years ago I was working renovating a house and a friend showed up with bear claw pastries to fuel our morning. I had already worked up a sweat, was half-starved anyway, and also wanted to be polite so I start eating one of the sugar-soaked, glazed, candy-pastries. I could barely get half of it down due to its overpowering sweetness. It felt like my mouth and throat were being coated in thick syrup that was making swallowing and breathing difficult. Try it yourself and see what I mean: avoid all sugar for twenty years than try to eat a bear claw. Go ahead - your throat will close up too!

Point of the story is that the donuts, cakes and candy you eat daily may be harder on your body than you realize. Most people think of just their belly fat or the number on the bathroom scale as a consequence of their eating habits. My opinion is that those things are trivial compared to the potential damage of over eating refined, artificial sweeteners. I have no problem with stevia as a sweetener, but for most applications, I believe nature provides us with honey for a reason.

Lastly, I avoid all fructose in the packaged food I buy. My understanding is that our bodies don't know what to do with fructose, so we store it as fat. Problem is that it is found in so many things from ketchup and salad dressing, fruit drinks, etc., so I do quite a lot of reading at the grocery store.

Here is my 'Things to Avoid' list, and quick explanation of why for each:

- Wheat gluten - drastically limit it. Breads and Wheat Thins are tasty, GF variations have dramatically improved in terms of taste and texture over the last ten years. Wheat products irritate my G.I. tract, are high carb and fattening. Besides, I would rather get my gluten and carbs from beer.

- Soy - feminizing, fattening (soybeans in natural form, aka edamame is okay). Soy products are as rule, highly processed.

- Sweets and refined sugar. Laboratory derived sweetener is a big NO. Embrace honey and stevia as your sweeteners.

- Basically, if it comes in a bag or a box, limit it to an occasional treat if you can. The food value is usually questionable, and their preservatives are a problem for the body.

- Between meal snacking - drink water with added electrolytes and see if that reduces cravings. Often we mistake the body asking for hydration as hunger or sugar cravings. I try to let my body do housekeeping between meals.

Pretty simple list, which is why I find it easy to follow. It happens to be more or less what my grandparents followed without having to think about it. These are things to shoot for over time. Old habits are tough to break when tackled suddenly, (remember my salt obsession?), but over time anything is do-able. If you have been eating coffee and doughnuts for 20 years, and you are thin and energetic, ignore my list! Otherwise, every other day eat eggs and coffee. Guilt is pointless and harmful. Enjoy what you eat but control it, don't let it control you.

The perfect diet is the diet on which you feel and perform your best.The diet that keeps you feeling full and without sugar spikes and mid-afternoon fatigue. If 20 cups of coffee, a salad and eggs and a Snickers works for you, than that's the perfect diet. Enjoy it! The good Dr. Kim would say that diet is only a twenty percent component of our overall health. This seems low to me but he repeated this often. He was, at the time, a 50 year old man with the body of a 25 year old, and was a multi-degree black belt in some martial art, the name of which escapes me. Point is, he practiced what he preached and was a model of health and fitness. Eat simply, seasonally and un-processed food as much as possible and keep moving. Movement is key. Movement is everything.

Supplement This

This is such a loaded subject for me, as I am sure it is for many other people seeking better health. I have spent a fortune on various supplements over the last forty years and the thing that strikes me about it all is what little difference it made in how I felt or performed. There are a couple of exceptions, which I will note, but the larger point I want to get across about what I have learned is that when it comes to diet and supplementation and even training, that **less is more**.

We spend so much time, effort and money on food, pills, powders, vitamins, etc., when for most people, certainly for me, the best 'medicine' is no medicine at all. Less food and fewer supplements means less stress on the body, more health and even longer life! I suggest you read about the benefits of daily fasting and autophagy if you want to understand where I am coming from on this. Check out this fascinating article from the US National Institutes of Health on autophagy: https://www.ncbi.nlm.nih.gov/pmc/articles/PMC3106288/ My very basic understanding of this is that by withholding food for extended periods, our bodies switch to a pure scavenging and house-keeping mode from which we derive substantial benefit.

We are brainwashed into thinking we need to stuff nutrition down our throats all day, but our bodies do just fine, and even thrive with less than we think, except for perhaps water and other fluids. I suggest spending your money on better food such as grass-fed beef and butter and avoid synthetic vitamins, which can actually be depleting your body of nutrients as it processes them! Ignore the marketing hype that is so rampant in the multi-billion dollar supplement industry.

I suggest experimenting with this by skipping breakfast and addressing your perceived hunger pangs by drinking water with added unsweetened lemon juice or other non-sweetened juice, or even a little bit of honey. You are in control, it is all conditioning and habit.

List of supplements I do take

- Cod liver oil - sweetened with lemon, preferably with no added vitamins - Omega-3 oils are excellent brain food
- I take an inexpensive digestive enzyme when I eat. I find this increasingly helpful as I get older as I never feel bloated or 'gassy' after eating.
- Zinc - but only when I feel a little 'puny', like when some half-wit with a cold coughs up a lung near me and I wake up with a sore throat the next morning.
- Electrolyte tablets - I put this in my water to replace the salts and other minerals lost through sweating.

Short list I will admit, but with the proper diet and omega-3 supplement, you are getting your nutrition, and are also addressing inflammation, which in my opinion, is what most people who suffer from illness, are really dealing with. Inflammation is the body's reaction to stress, whether from some internal dysfunction or from behavioral things like over-eating and over-training. Reduce and avoid inflammation and live better. Food, drink, work, play, everything in moderation.

Inversion Table - You Need One

One thing I notice about many of the men of all ages I meet is how common back problems are among them. Women, either by design or behavior, seem to be relatively immune from this. I feel very fortunate to have avoided this malady but would like to know whether this is due to genetics or dumb luck, since I want to avoid the misery and limitation that comes with having a 'bad back'. Although I am active, I also tend to sit for extended periods at my desk, and I understand the importance of posture and holding my spine straight and all that.

I remember reading that even when you are laying down flat on our back, that the spine is experiencing a 25 percent retraction. Other words, our muscles and connective tissue exert pressure on the spinal column, even when the affect of gravity is removed. If only there was an easy way to temporarily eliminate all pressure from the spine and even subject it to negative pressure.

Just so happens there is a way to do this, its called an **inversion table**, and over the years it has been a game-changer for me.

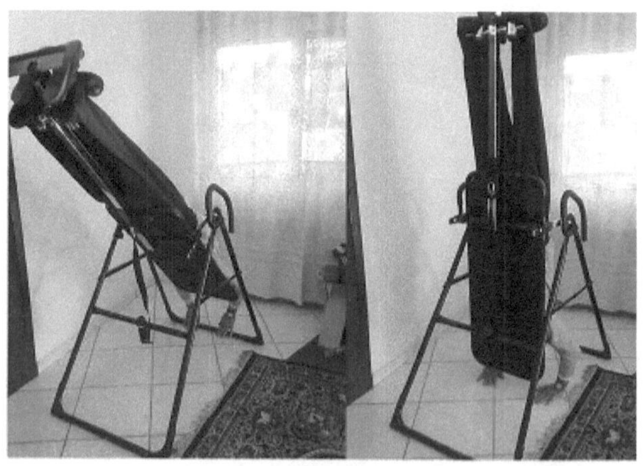

This is something you want to start with in a very deliberate and careful way. Simply put, you step into the table, bind your feet or ankles, then gently push backward and allow the table to pivot in the center which brings your feet up over your head while you hang vertically. My table happens to be made by Nordictrac and it allows me to completely hang, bat-like, for as long as I want. I find that my feet and ankles are my limiting factor; after about ten minutes they start to feel a little uncomfortable so I swing back to start position. Wearing thick athletic socks allows me to significantly prolong this excellent, hard-tissue exercise.

When you use an inversion table the first time, you likely want to stop at 60 or so degrees rather than going all-in and swinging into the full vertical. Your system needs several brief sessions to acclimate to the very unique stress you are introducing with this machine. Some people, for whatever reason, cannot tolerate the 'upside-down' feeling and sadly, never give this movement a fair chance. Even if you are 'that' person, if you pace yourself and work incrementally, you will soon get used to the disorientation and might even start to enjoy the feeling and related benefits of hanging upside down.

Whenever I feel any kind of soreness in my back, usually from weekend warrior-type activity, I turn to my inversion table for a session or two, a couple of days apart. The force of gravity decompresses my spine and creates a negative pressure between bone and cartilage that literally pulls in fluid and nutrients and accelerates repair and recovery. The benefits are immediate and long term. Back soreness, especially in the lower back seems to magically disappear within a few minutes.

Like everything else, too much of a good thing, in this case too much inversion time, has also made me a bit sore, although this went away after a short period of time - usually 3 or 4 hours. I have found that brief, ten minute or so sessions are perfect for the recovery and maintenance of my back.

You can get some of the benefits of the inversion table by simply grabbing and hanging from a pull-up bar. The back-stretch this provides is definitely beneficial, however unless you have world-class grip strength, or some clever way to take the stress off your hands and forearms, you won't be hanging that way for long, too many small muscles are involved in hanging using the hands, whereas the inversion table is really about hard tissue exercise. Besides, nothing approaches the efficiency of the inversion table at pulling or stretching apart the spine.

Look for an inversion table deal where you can try it out and return it if you hate it. I would bet that for the vast majority of you, if you give it a month of careful evaluation, and several brief sessions of no more than five minutes each per week, you will be hooked and will use and rely forever on this wonderful machine.

Are You Falling Asleep Again!?

Sleep is so important that we devote a big chunk of our lives to it. Funny how things change, including even something as fundamental as sleep, as we move through the phases of life. I have a typical sleep profile for a man my age with an intact prostate. I find it ridiculously easy to fall asleep, it truly is as if I have a bubble level inside my skull that switches my consciousness off whenever I tilt my head far enough to move the bubble to one side. I can drink a strong cup of black coffee at 8pm, with my signature, three heaping spoonsful of Folgers Crystals, and be out like a light right on the couch where I finished it at 8:15pm. Caffeine is no match for the bubble level.

So, I eventually find myself in bed but now I am working through my overnight routine. This means bathroom trips every two hours until 6am where, usually out of mild annoyance, I get up and, of course, head to the bathroom. I must say that the elderly do get their money's worth from the plumbing.

Falling asleep is child's play for me, whereas staying asleep is the real challenge. It isn't that I even need as much sleep as I did as a kid, but I do need a good six or so hours. I can tell by the following afternoon if I need sleep and I will usually execute a 5 or 10 minute power nap - which is something I highly recommend. More on that in a bit.

Sleep is also an area where women seem to be wired better for it, and my wild guess is that this is a big reason why women tend to live longer than men. That and the fact that women seem to stay physically and mentally more active and engaged in the later years, but when you stop and think about it, that could also be related to their better sleep proficiency as well.

There are a few things I have found that help me stay asleep for longer stretches at night, which translates to more energy, better recall and mental ability the next day and a better sense of well-being.

Here are my recommendations for better sleep:

- Cease all fluid intake after 8pm (unless of course I am goofing with friends over beers, life is short - don't judge)

- Turn on a white noise machine at very low volume, just enough to hear it, not drown out the world.

- Use a blanket - I have always liked to be cool when I sleep, but I have found that being a little on the warm side means I get up less frequently to urinate.

- Drink alcohol less often - I used to have a couple beers after work most days (every day?). Now I wait until the weekend and thus drink much less overall. Alcohol seems to irritate my system and bladder enough to cause frequent bathroom visits, so eliminating it during the week allows me to sleep longer and better.

Of course, working to maintain overall health and conditioning has a huge impact on better sleep. Just by virtue of being lucky enough to avoid illness and disease all contribute to what should be our natural ability to enjoy restful, healthy sleep. But what happens when stress, an argument, work deadline, or other problem interferes with sleep and drags you down the following day?

This is what the power nap is for!

Power napping is something I remember hearing about from President Jimmy Carter of all people. Yes, that's how old I am. This was back in the 70's, and, because I was a late teen at the time, I thought it was odd that anyone could benefit from a ten minute nap, and anyway it was probably pointless, just like everything else about his administration. Snap!

Here is the thing I have since learned about the power nap; when done a certain way, it is an amazing performance tool. No kidding!

The real secret of the power nap for me is keeping it short and sweet. By short, I'm talking ten or maybe fifteen minutes, but five minutes is enough, it really depends on whether or not I lose consciousness. Other words, I allow myself to drift off to sleep, but just for five or ten minutes, and then I somehow wake up and am suddenly back in the game but feeling energized and alert. It's the strangest thing, but it works.

I spend a lot of time driving in rural Florida, and there is the occasional day where I find myself working at staying alert and fighting that drowsy feeling. (Hello Geico people - please skip this section!) This problem always strikes in the afternoon following a night of poor sleep or perhaps an extra early wake-up call. I used to fight it, and sometimes still do depending on what is happening on a given day. But, when I have fifteen minutes to spare, I look for a quiet, shaded spot and execute the power nap.

I am lucky to have reclining seats that go almost flat. I always wear a hat of some kind which is a convenient eye covering during my nap. Florida is too warm about 9 months out of the year to nap in the car without the air conditioning running, which means the engine is on, but this and the A/C fan is really a perfect white noise machine. Sometimes I feel I am re-creating a running car ambiance in my bedroom in order to better sleep.

By the way, in August when it's 102 degrees and 90% humidity and the weather people are advising us to stay indoors, I will usually pop the hood and raise it a little, like you sometimes see the cops do when their cruisers are parked and running. This allows a ton more heat dissipation from the engine.

So there I am, fully reclined with my hat pulled down over my face. Engine is idling with cool air blowing on low, radio off and cellphone volume very low. The drowsy feeling I have been fighting for the last hour or so is now allowed to wash over me and before I know it, the bubble level is switching my brain to neutral and then off.

Whether due to environment, location, engine miss, I have no idea, but within five to fifteen minutes later, I wake up. The feeling of alertness and renewal is difficult to believe or describe. It seems to be the act of drifting into momentary unconsciousness that provides the boost, rather than the duration of the nap itself. I rarely take a proper afternoon nap, but an hour or two on the rack at home usually leaves me feeling groggy and sluggish for extended periods after waking. Not so at all with the power nap, whose affects are immediate and invigorating. This tactic has never failed to carry me through the rest of the day in proper form.

Alcohol and Drugs

I struggled with this topic for awhile because after all, this is a training guide for long term health, not an anti-drug and alcohol thesis.

I want you to know where I stand, which, based on experience and observation, makes me somewhat libertarian when it comes to this subject. I find it fascinating that a hundred or so years ago, the local drugstore stocked things like opiates and soda containing cocaine, whereas now, many previously benign cold remedies are locked away behind the counter and you must consult with the pharmacist if you need a Sudafed. What happened to us man?

Anything that impairs your performance, changes your trajectory as you travel through life. I have yet to find someone who enjoyed a higher sustained performance level through the use of alcohol or drugs, although I am not so naive as to doubt such a person exists, I would view that person as the exception that proves the rule anyway.

Those with a compulsion to drink or take recreational drugs to get through the day are in real trouble on a lot of levels, their health being just one of them. I once knew a man who was quite talented in his trade, despite his habit of drinking at least a fifth (back then a quart, actually) of cheap whiskey each and every day, starting with his first glass over breakfast. The first thing he did after waking up was take a big vomit. This was twenty years ago and I have lost touch with him. But imagine what 7300 bottles of whiskey have done to his liver and brain since then! This is the number, at one per day, he is likely to have drunk over this time.

Point is, the body is an amazing recovery machine. We throw tons of pollutants at ourselves and I am always surprised at how much it withstands. Still, it is safe to assume that he has accelerated the aging process and made things much harder for himself than if he had been able to moderate his drinking.

I have a neighbor of sixteen years who for the entire time has been a heavy tweaker. His methamphetamine habit has gotten worse and more obvious with each passing year. He is manic and schizophrenic at this point, (my layman's opinion), and even his facial structure is changing which is likely because his teeth have rotted away from his chronic dry mouth. He has become unreachable in any meaningful way. His entire life appears to revolve around obtaining and taking more Meth. My opinion is that only a period of prolonged incarceration will save his life, which may be too late since he must be mid-forties by now.

Point is, without getting too philosophical here, these people have always existed.

You will pass by lots of them on the side of the road as you travel through your life. Some you can help but most you cannot. I have tried repeatedly and failed, simply because they don't want help, they want more drugs or alcohol. It matters little what I think about it or them, but I know I want to avoid becoming like them. I would rather live my life free from the shackles of that kind of intense dependency.

Doctors and Other Drug Dealers

I feel I must at least mention the medical profession again as it relates to the subject of drugs. My opinion is that one of the few things for which a doctor is truly useful, pain relief, is just the thing he or she is least likely to provide.

I know people who live with chronic, un-ending pain, and I have learned that evil can be best described simply as chronic pain. It would be great if we had a modern medical industry that developed treatments that helped people instead of fleeced them. Humanity desperately needs a machine or process that measures pain and provides a way to switch it off. We seem to be too concerned with the affects of nicotine on mosquitoes and whether polar bears can be gay to have the time to tackle life's real problems.

How about a national effort to target and solve chronic pain? Offer enough incentives so that kids clamor to become neurobiologists or whatever it takes and solve this! Drugs that stop pain without the high or addiction so people can return to work and have a life. Let's work on that.

My observation, based on substantial experience dealing with our medical-industrial complex over the past twenty five plus years, is that you can accurately measure how screwed you are in life by determining how dependent you have become on doctors for your well-being,

I don't put all blame on doctors for this, the insurance industry with their cost-shifting, direct payments to doctors and indecipherable fee schedules, as well as governmental oversight malpractice has created this morass. Doctors, for their part are basically small business owners first, with payroll, rent, suppliers and so forth, taking their time and energy. Their patients, as customers, are absolutely terrible! These sick, needy people don't even pay their doctor anymore, the insurance company does. .

I used to look for doctors who did not accept insurance. Without exception, their offices were quiet, with a small group of very professional, experienced medical professionals, and the level of care was acceptable. Today, the first thing the average practice wants to know is with whom are you insured. There are usually up to a dozen, surly, under-paid clerks processing mountains of reports and forms to keep the insurance and governmental gravy flowing. We patients have become an obstacle to them; an inevitable speed bump on their receivables highway. The slightest inconvenience we cause is met with anger and shame. The government and insurance industry created this problem, doctors played along. Lexus and lake house payments must be made.

Judging by the attitudes on display there, patients are nothing more than hoops of liability that doctors must jump through on their way to the money. There is plenty of blame to go around for this.

Please understand that I am not an advocate for single payer, medicaid for all, socialist nonsense. Those at the top who advocate for that would never allow themselves or their families to live within such a system. Moving from the private insurance-based system that has ruined medical care to a government only system is the only possible way we could worsen the situation.

What we need is every doctor, surgeon, lab, clinic and hospital competing for our business. We need transparency and competition. We need the government to protect us from bad doctors and insane prices, and doctors from predatory lawyers. We need insurance that reimburses us for our medical expenses, and while we're at it, make it a crime for an insurance clerk to discuss our treatment, condition and medical expenses with anyone from the medical community. Lastly, this business of doctors making us jump through hoops to get records and share *our* information with us and with those we request must stop, immediately. Doctors openly and readily share any shred of data requested by a nameless and faceless insurance clerk or governmental official requesting it- because that is who pays them! The rules for us, usually based on mis-quoted HIPAA law, are quite different and are used as a barrier and an excuse to refuse to help. We don't write the check, after all, so why should a doctor go out of his way to give us a test result?

Notice how politicians never mention any of these real, ongoing problems. They provide sound bite ready solutions, which are anything but. My question to them has to be: how does being shut out of the doctor-insurance company process and replacing that with being shut out of the doctor-medicare- for-all process provide any relief for the great unwashed?

We need a return to the system my grandparents had!

Have you ever watched a medical show like Doc Martin? This was a hit English show whose main character was a village doctor, a brilliant general practitioner, who saw patients either at the clinic connected to his home, or, when needed, wherever they were.

This is a modern show so I am lead to believe that this is somewhat taken as standard medical care over there. What strikes me about the show is how effective one doctor can be when he or she takes responsibility for the whole person, and conversely, how over-specialized our medical profession is and therefore how under-served we are. Additionally, with over-specialization has come wild duplication of expenses and thus premiums, as well as significant time delays in getting proper treatment and relief. Making matters worse, our government enacts laws like HIPAA, as a feel-good patients rights move, but which is used by medical people as a barrier to keep us from our own records, and records sharing between doctors to a minimum.

Basically, any actual 'health care' in such an overwrought system is purely a coincidence.

Should you be in need of a doctor to get a fracture cared for, or laceration stitched up, rejoice! We have great systems in place for these things. Treatments for diseases of the immune system, neuropathy, psychiatry and so many others means you are dealing with a pre-modern understanding of these issues and a greedy, broken delivery system. Find alternate treatment paths if at all possible. The medical system as it exists in its present form should be consulted as a last, rather than first resort, if quality of life and mental health are your top priorities.

Just give me healthcare that is half as good as my dogs receive at the vet. That's all I ask, which is apparently too much. Avoid all medication (okay insulin is one of a few exceptions) requiring long-term or permanent use. Drugs kill, unless your MD prescribes them, then drugs kill with FDA approval. There are usually alternatives to the chemicals being pushed by your doctor that are also less harmful to you. Your doctor will vehemently disagree for several stated reasons that are all in-the-box thinking and safe for him. Then, he will prescribe stuff that can cause grave problems or at least make you feel worse than before you began treatment and basically experiment on you. It has become a lousy, dangerous, unaffordable system.

Everything in moderation, including drugs and alcohol, and especially doctors.

We are all Mental

"Obstacles do not block the path, they are the path" -unknown

As with the other sections of this book, everything I have learned about how our brains work as we age, I've picked up through observation. My relatives provided early examples, both good and bad, of the aging process, and interestingly, my dogs have also contributed much to my understanding of how this all works, at least for the vast majority of us.

I believe that brain health is by far the primary factor of our overall health. I once had a pretty little dog named Rosie. Rosie was a tough, independent-minded little thing who made us laugh every day for over seventeen years. I would take her for regular checkups, including her last one at age seventeen, and the vet would say things like, "They should all be this healthy, at any age".

Then one day, a very sad thing happened. Rosie gave me a look that made me think she had no idea who I was. She began the process of retreating into her head, and would sometimes be terrified of my wife and me. I would often have to corner her outside and catch her to bring her in. It was heartbreaking because she had no idea who we were and seemed to be panicky to get back to familiar territory.

Almost as soon as her dementia began, her extraordinarily healthy body began a rapid decline. Within a few months, she would suffer a heart attack and then a couple of strokes and we had to end her suffering.

Rosie was part of a pattern I have witnessed since childhood about brains and aging. She reinforced my understanding that no matter how healthy we are, eventually it is our time to leave this plane of existence.

But, Rosie lived a long life and right up to the end, she was physically capable and pain free. I'll take that any day over languishing in a bed being tended to for basic needs until I draw my final breath. I think you would too.

You need to pay attention to brain health at some point, and begin to nourish this vital organ. By this I mean providing it the fats and omega oils it needs through diet and supplementation, avoiding harmful affects of being sedentary and other oxygen restrictive things such as excessive smoking. Simply stated; a healthy body requires a healthy brain and vice verse. We need to exercise the brain too, unless we no longer need it - which is never!

A healthy brain means you also must keep yourself in learning mode. Being social is one way to keep synapses firing, but acquiring new skills, reading, hobbies and being otherwise mentally stimulated are important components when it comes to mental and brain health. Sure, memory becomes less reliable over time, but there are excellent exercises available via mp3 you can play while driving to exercise your recall 'muscle' and keep your brain in learning mode.

You or I may have a genetic ticking time-bomb as far as our brain function is concerned. Even so, making the most of our God-given ability and time we do have are main components of health and happiness.

Relationship Advice From a Loner

We seem to all be wired differently, but are also connected in some enigmatic way. I consider myself somewhat of a loner; quite content to be by myself for extended periods with only my thoughts as company. Being alone feels like a luxury to me. I can think and do what I want without worrying about those around me. You may feel the same way, or you may find this unimaginable, and quickly feel lonely and isolated without constant human companionship.

The challenge for me is to embrace those with personalities so different from mine, and even to celebrate those differences. Sure, people can be frustrating and angering, treacherous and at times even dangerous. My mom taught me to see the good in people, and almost everyone I've ever met had some positive trait. Problem is that many people, including myself, often present a public image, a protective coating if you will, that must by navigated with a certain amount of time and patience, before the genuine article is revealed. This is what is interesting about human interaction and relationships.

My advice about people is that everyone has a story and some knowledge from which we can benefit, if we are willing to invest some time and energy. The connection we have with others can be demonstrated by the joy we receive when we help them. We seem to be wired to be at our best when we help and learn from one another, which lends credibility to the idea of a creator and intelligent design.

My point here is that I struggle with the idea of being engaged with my fellow man, because my natural tendency is to live alone in a cave. But my mental health and longevity are dependent on my willingness to stay involved with others, to help them and be helped by them. Sure, there are setbacks and regrets throughout the journey - oh are there ever! But there are many more benefits and victories and even elation that comes with human companionship and relationships.

Stay involved with people, even if you are bruised from past relationships and would rather go it alone. Should you be physically isolated and can engage only through email and websites, great! The internet is nothing if not a phenomenal communication tool. Your mental health, your brain health and well-being depend on it. Depression is a waste of precious time. Find someone or a group you can relate to. You are not unique! Everyone has baggage and someone needs your help. Find them and connect with them and everyone benefits.

Final Thoughts

One thing I have noticed about life is how my priorities have evolved over time. Most young people eventually discover the freedom of accepting their own physical limits and looks as the trivia they are, and begin to focus instead on deeper issues such as career and family. Sure, it is certainly possible to develop the physique of a Stallone or Rock, and if doing so is where your passion is, I applaud you. Most people would be happy just enjoying the health and stamina that comes with a certain minimum attention to detail regarding their eating and exercising habits.

For me, the task of working out to achieve pure stud level status gave way to the pressures of life that we all face. But the trick there, in my opinion, is to preserve a tiny, one percent sliver of time for the physical exercises that serve us so well as we work and perform in the remaining ninety nine percent.

I also know that you can bring about drastic change in your health and well-being by taking the smallest incremental steps in the right direction. If you are thirty pounds overweight, the last thing you want to do is go on a diet. Instead, you want to introduce healthier food into your daily routine, which means less processed food with its fattening preservatives and sugar. Eating less or less often is much more difficult than eating better food. Ramping up your physical activity very slowly while eating a little smarter will accelerate your progress toward feeling better, having more energy and fuel your desire to tackle more challenges. Your success will 'feed' on itself, spurring you on to stay more active, eat increasingly better and so on. Just don't go overboard with any of it and drive yourself or those around you, nuts.

I once knew a man, an executive working for a large company, who was a true fitness fanatic. He had the amusing habit of handing back the restaurant menu to the server and would proceed to dictate every ingredient, spice, cooking method etc, he expected them to execute. I can appreciate this, but the time and effort it required were challenging, to say the least. Then, immediately after the meal, usually just outside in front of the restaurant, he would execute and hold a handstand. For several minutes!

This was, he claimed, a secret to better digestion. Somewhere today, as I write this, that crazy bastard is probably holding a handstand. The point is, and always will be: everything in moderation, don't be a fanatic, your body is forgiving, just work with its natural abilities, which are formidable. We did not evolve in such a way that inverting ourselves following meals was necessary, let alone beneficial.

If it strikes you as odd, or worse, it probably is.

I try to remember that so much of life is just a game we play with ourselves, and in the process, often drive ourselves to distraction. You could eat only cotton candy for a week and little will change within that small period of time. Same for salad, or celery which is what makes this difficult for us and our need for the quick payoff. *There is no quick payoff.* The good things in life take time, which is probably how it should be.

The best way past that is to define a specific goal and measure your progress against that instead of some nebulous thing like whether you see a change in the mirror or on the bathroom scale. Set a goal of something like, before noon eating fruit or water only and no food after eight at night and no snacking between lunch and dinner for a month. Write that down and do it. After a month, you will have ingrained that as a habit and you will have already begun to notice positive changes in yourself. I promise.

Tony Robbins once said this:

"This is the secret to happiness in one word: Progress. Progress equals happiness. That's because reaching a goal is satisfying, but only temporarily so. When you reach the next level of 'making it', you realize that when you get there, you'll see another level".

How true that is! Sure, reaching goals is exhilarating, but we soon begin to experience the feeling of 'ok, so what's next'? The real fun is in the reaching, the struggle. The end, the goal, can be anti-climatic compared to the effort put forth to reach it. Human nature is a wonderful and often mysterious thing. Embrace the struggle, hang on and enjoy the ride.

I appreciate you for choosing this book. I hope it serves you well and maybe provides a fresh perspective on your health as you move forward through life.

Never forget the words of C.S. Lewis:

"You can't go back and change the beginning, but you can start where you are and change the ending"

My only question is; what are you waiting for, an engraved invitation? Keep moving!

The End

Me, Myself, and Why

I am, judging from the images and messages received daily from our youth oriented pop-culture, at age 59, a very old man. Apparently, its a wonder I can still drive or remember my address, but somehow I do.

I am neither a sports doctor, nor professional athlete. In fact, I am physically quite average in looks, stature, height, weight etc. My weight is within 15 pounds of what it was at age 18 when I got out of high school. I do believe that most of my weight gain is muscle weight, although I'm sure that I now have a slightly higher body fat percentage than I did back then.

Also know that I care little about these things and I'm only sharing this to give you some perspective about what you have read. I have personal experience, although second hand, living with chronic illness and pain and I am here to tell you that you can easily define evil by thinking of it in terms of illness and pain. Especially when those things happen to a young person as it has to my family. Your health and feeling of well-being are priceless gifts, but are also, sadly, things that we take for granted until (hopefully never for you) they are lost.

I have learned a thing or two along the way since my days of playing baseball, football, or basketball all day, every day in the steamy summers of Florida. Much of what I wanted to tell you I learned the hard way, through trial and error. There is so much information available on the subject of health, fitness and diet that it is very easy to get loaded down and over-think these things. Doing so often leads to feelings of being overwhelmed and an analysis paralysis.

I want you to avoid all that. The reality is that you win when you keep it very simple, do what has to be done, then get back into your real (non-gym) life! Ultimately, this book is what works and has worked for me and it is, therefore, my opinion. I have tried many exercise and fitness methods, routines and diets over the years and eventually discovered, developed really, what to take from all that and apply to myself. I suggest you take what I have to say and do the same thing; find your own best way forward, but armed with the knowledge and perspective of others who have approached these same issues and had similar questions. We all learn and benefit from each other, and we must strive to be open to new information and advice. My view is that to be truly 'old' is to be intolerant of new ideas. Simple as that. To be so set in our ways and beliefs that a new perspective on any subject is annoying and must be summarily rejected and dismissed.

Let's resolve right here to never be that guy!

I sincerely hope you found something in this guide to help you on your journey. Given the fact that you are reading self improvement material in the first place means we share common interests and priorities. I have witnessed people around me lose their health and mobility and frankly, it scares the hell out of me. I have learned to appreciate my God-given gift of health and durability and want to preserve it. I know you do too, who wouldn't?

I would be forever grateful if you would leave me a review on Amazon, unless of course you despised the book, in that case, please heed the words of my Mom, "If you can't say anything nice, don't say anything at all." If only the world operated by Mom's rules, am I right?

Thank you again, and I wish you good health and boundless energy.

Mike